THE SMILES BEHIND THE MASK

Volume 2

Celebrating
30 Years of Publishing
in India

Other Books in the Series

The Smiles Behind the Mask, Volume 1

THE SMILES BEHIND THE MASK

Volume 2

Heartwarming Stories from

Apollo Hospitals

HarperCollins *Publishers* India

First published in India by HarperCollins *Publishers* 2023
4th Floor, Tower A, Building No. 10, DLF Cyber City,
DLF Phase II, Gurugram, Haryana – 122002
www.harpercollins.co.in

2 4 6 8 10 9 7 5 3 1

P-ISBN: 978-93-5699-795-0
E-ISBN: 978-93-5699-793-6

Typeset in 11/15.2 Bell MT at
Manipal Technologies Limited, Manipal

Printed and bound at
Thomson Press (India) Ltd

We dedicate this collection to our valued patients, with grateful thanks for the trust they place in us, and with the promise that we shall continue to do our best for them, always…

Contents

THE STORIES

Foreword

'Wherever the art of medicine is loved, there is also a love of humanity.'

– Hippocrates the Great

WHEN A PERSON IS WHEELED INTO A HOSPITAL, THEIR entire family and loved ones are swinging between hope and despair. While only the patient must go through their journey of healing, the medical staff in attendance can and must do their best to make that path easier, through kind thought and positive action.

At Apollo Hospitals, we have always lived by the belief that a patient is much more than just an infirm body. And that their mental and emotional well-being contribute immensely to their physical recovery. Through our thirty-nine years of existence, our amazing staff have proved time and time again that little deeds of kindness and small gestures of thoughtfulness are worth their weight in gold.

While it is not possible to record or reward each of these heartwarming episodes, we are delighted to present to you this short collection of fifty stories that celebrate our warriors. Each narrative will restore your faith in human goodness and bring a smile to your face.

Our eternal gratitude to Dr Prathap C. Reddy, our founder and chairman, for inspiring us to go the extra mile and showing us the true meaning of healing.

Dr Preetha Reddy
Shobana Kamineni
Suneeta Reddy
Dr Sangita Reddy
Hyderabad
25 December 2022

Story 1

Healing with Knitting

Apollo Super Speciality Hospital, Noida

IN THE SCORCHING HEAT OF JUNE 2018, WHEN EVERYONE ELSE was fighting the blazing sun, Sonakshi Rana was hit with the searing diagnosis of rectal cancer. She was put under the care of Dr Manish and Dr Krutali at Apollo Hospitals, Noida.

Though she was coping bravely with the trauma of chemotherapy, it wasn't easy for her emotionally. Her greatest anxiety was for her family, and what they would be going through because of her condition. With each passing day, she found herself feeling more vulnerable and drained. Just when she seemed to be losing all hope, Apollo staff members Ms Shabnam and Mr Sajesh decided to lift her out of the depression.

During one of Sonakshi's chemotherapy sessions, they gifted her a knitting set. She was a little taken aback because her knitting skills were zero. However, she took it as a blessing, and with the help of the staff, mastered the art of knitting within no time. This new skill proved to be a wonderful distraction from her cycle of pain. Soon enough, Sonakshi's hands began to play magic with the needles. She knitted three sweaters, eight hats and five pairs of socks, and believe it or not, started looking forward to her chemotherapy sessions. On each visit, she brought a knitted return gift for the staff.

In 2022, the last day of her chemotherapy dawned. She had been awaiting this moment for a long time but choked up when saying goodbye to those who had looked after her. As a parting gift, she presented them with a beautiful red sweater that she had designed and knit herself. They say one act of kindness leads to another, and Sonakshi's act of gratitude keeps inspiring the staff to support their patients, day after day.

Story 2

Facing it with Confidence

Apollo Hospitals, Jubilee Hills, Hyderabad

THE YEAR 2022 CHANGED A LOT OF THINGS FOR MALISA Phiri Zulu. A resident of Zambia, Malisa was brought to Apollo Hospitals, Jubilee Hills in January 2022 and treated for laryngeal cancer under Dr Umanath Nayak, head and neck oncologist. After the surgery, a tracheostomy tube became a part of her permanently. It showed as a large lump right beneath her Adam's apple, and the thought of facing her colleagues and society back in Zambia began to haunt her.

Conscious of her appearance, Malisa tried everything she could to look presentable and avoid being commented on. She cloaked herself behind scarves and shawls, and tried her best to communicate clearly, even though her voice emerged as a bare whisper. When she visited India for a review, it was apparent that she was struggling to maintain her looks and dignity and had lost her zest for life. This was when Nurse Sandhya Isaac, the international patient coordinator, and Usha Prabhakar, the chief nursing officer of Apollo, Telangana region, stepped up to help her.

Ms Usha and a few of her staff members designed beautiful scarves adorned with laces and crochet in different colours to match Malisa's attire. The scarves even had gauze pads to ensure that the material would not hurt the tube and prevent any dust particles from spreading infection. This act of kindness brought a smile on Malisa's face. She was discharged in March 2022, and she left the hospital with her head held high.

Just a small gesture can make all the difference to a person's self-esteem and spirits. And a hospital is one place where it means even more to patients battling life's greatest challenges. For this understanding and compassion, Apollo staff deserve kudos!

Story 3

His Healing Heroes

Apollo Hospitals, Jubilee Hills, Hyderabad

JUST WHEN HIS LONG-AWAITED DREAM OF CO-DIRECTING A movie for Nani (lead actor) was about to come true, his world of dreams and the real world collapsed for Roshan Das. An only son in the family and a young emerging co-director, his life was shattered when he was brought in an unconscious state to Apollo Hospitals, Jubilee Hills, Hyderabad in October 2021. He had been diagnosed with cardioembolic stroke, that is, dilated cardiomyopathy, under

Dr Manoj K. Agarwal, senior consultant cardiologist. The condition had left half of his body completely paralysed.

The stroke had left him fragmented, both emotionally and physically, and his life came to a standstill. He went into a deep depression and simply refused to respond to any treatment or physiotherapy. This was the time when the hospital's consultant neurologist, Dr Sandeep Nayani, paramedic staff members and nursing staff, including Nurse Sandhya and Akul Bhavani, stepped in as guiding angels for him. They decided to bring back the enthusiasm in him with the things that mattered to him the most—films—and most importantly, acting with Nani. The patient had a heartfelt desire to make a film with Nani as the lead actor and had been waiting for a good story to pick when he had this health issue.

The hospital team started creating different collages, putting together pictures from his stronger days, along with the actors that performed in his movies in consort. They motivated him and tried to surprise him every day with various crusades. While he was unable to move or talk, gradually his eyes came to life and spoke his heart out. Seeing a positive response from Roshan, the staff even arranged visits from his supporters and the people close to his heart.

All this time, while the staff was trying hard to infuse the zeal back into him, his family, especially his mother and sister, were going through a hard time dealing with the anxiety and shock. Seeing the staff's efforts for Roshan, the family also raised their faith. Soon the endeavours bore results and after twenty-five struggling days, Roshan was discharged in November 2021. The nurses, doctors and everyone that had helped him during those terrifying days could clearly see the happiness that Roshan was trying to convey through his beaming eyes. His gratitude for helping him come back to normal life was the staff's unmeasurable reward and another step towards facilitating healthy, happy lives at Apollo.

Story 4

We Care, Baby

Apollo BGS Hospitals, Mysuru

IN 2021, ONE-YEAR-OLD AASIF WAS BROUGHT TO APOLLO Hospitals, Mysuru with a history of ulcers. Under Paediatric Gastroenterologist Dr Athira, the little one went through a surgical process to remove pus formation in his rectum. Post-surgery, the baby lost his appetite and could not digest whatever he was fed. His parents and grandmother were in unbearable torment.

This was when Sister Prema, in charge of the ward and herself a mother of two, came to the rescue. Learning the medical history of Aasif, she did some research and concluded that feeding the baby ragi seri, a type of traditional food, might help. The cereal is fed to babies between the age of zero to three years. One of her staff members had recently returned from her maternity leave, and Sister Prema asked her to prepare a bowl of ragi seri, with the help of Mr Ravi and Mr Viswanath of the food and beverages department, adding in lots of nuts, ghee and love.

As soon as Aasif saw the bowl of ragi seri, his eyes beamed with excitement, and to everyone's surprise, the staff was able to feed him the full bowl in no time. Seeing their little bundle of joy eat, the parents and the grandmother were really happy and thanked Sister Prema a million times. Gradually, the baby recovered.

Upon discharge, the parents personally thanked the sister for her motherly care. Even now, when Aasif comes for a routine check-up every three months, he always meets Sister Prema. These small little gestures reinforce Apollo's belief that 'little things can make a big difference.'

Story 5

Where There Is a Will

Apollo Hospitals, Navi Mumbai

BALJEET SINGH WAS DIAGNOSED WITH LUMBAR CANAL stenosis with neurogenic claudication in August 2022 at Apollo Hospitals, Navi Mumbai. He was admitted to the hospital and advised surgical management by Dr Sunil Kutti. During his stay at the hospital staff members Mehrin and Navjeet became closely attached to Baljeet and his wife and were a constant source of comfort to the couple.

Initially, Baljeet refused to undergo the surgery. With his advancing age, he feared that he might not survive the surgery and might never be able to see his four sons again, all settled in the US. But it is rightly said, 'Where there is a will, there is a way.'

After multiple counselling sessions and the firm support of his wife, Mehrin and Navjeet, Baljeet finally agreed to the surgery. It was a tough decision for him. To make things slightly easier for him, Mehrin and Navjeet, along with the other staff members, gave him a little surprise. Chef Pranjal from the pantry prepared a special cake for him which had 'Get Well Soon' written on top; and a video call was also arranged with all his four sons. Shortly before the procedure, he spoke to his sons and entered the operation theatre with a contented heart.

The surgery was successful, and while he was under observation, Navjeet read out the Mul Mantra path to him, a Sikh prayer for health, every morning. In a short time, Baljeet was back to his happy, optimistic self, and repeatedly praised the doctors and nursing staff. He even hosted a lunch gathering for the entire team that had attended on him, as a small token of gratitude and love. Baljeet is doing well now and is still in touch with Mehrin and Navjeet. Even today, his voice is heavy with emotion when he thanks the staff for treating him like a family member.

Story 6

Caring Like a Son

Apollo Hospitals, Navi Mumbai

ADMITTED TO APOLLO HOSPITALS, NAVI MUMBAI IN December 2021 for bilateral total knee replacement under Dr Siddharth Yadav, Ragini Devi, sixty-eight, and her husband were nervous and a bit overwhelmed. Their son resided in the US and could not make it for the surgery. Though Ragini's husband was attending to her every need, they were an elderly couple and needed much more than each other's company.

A runner named Krishna was given the responsibility to shift Ragini to the operation theatre for surgery. He formed a close bond with Ragini during this short window of time. She remarked that he reminded her of her son, and even Krishna dutifully cared for her as her own. With him beside them, the couple's anxiety transformed into hope and assurance. The surgery was successful, and during recovery, Krishna was there for her throughout.

Gradually, Ragini Devi got the green signal to be discharged from the hospital. Though the guest relations executive (GRE) was supporting and helpful in every way, Ragini's husband was still a bit disoriented and in low spirits. Once again, Krishna came to their rescue. Despite his day off, he immediately volunteered to help. He got in touch with the third party administrator desk, informed the GRE and took the entire responsibility of getting Ragini discharged in his hands.

While leaving the hospital, Ragini, with an emotional heart and a tearful eye, specially mentioned Krishna's efforts to the higher management. She suggested that unselfish gestures like those of Krishna should be well-acknowledged and rewarded. Ragini is hale and hearty now, living a healthy life.

Story 7

The Unlocking

Apollo Hospitals, Navi Mumbai

In August 2022, eight-year-old Noor Khan was brought to the emergency ward of Apollo Hospitals, Navi Mumbai in the late hours of the night. Noor's index finger was stuck in a cylindrical lock. The entire emergency team was trying every possible way to relieve Noor of her pain, but no technique seemed to work.

With every slipping second, her agony was becoming unbearable, and her parents were growing desperate. While on his normal night rounds, Santosh Lanka noticed the chaos in the emergency. Usually, this hour of the night was quiet, so he asked a nurse and found out about Noor's situation.

With permission from the clinical team, he examined Noor's hand. Though everyone had almost given up, Noor's mother was still clinging on to the last bit of hope, her eyes closed in prayer. Santosh gently held Noor's hand and skilfully moved it left and right, displaying expertise. There was pin-drop silence, with every eye on Santosh. While everyone was confused about what Santosh was trying to do, he ingeniously freed the little girl's finger from the lock, with minimal bruising.

Noor's mother was the first one to break the silence, offering her gratitude to the Almighty and to Santosh. Soon, the entire emergency team joined the mother in applauding Santosh's efforts. Noor's father, who was too overwhelmed to speak for a while, finally spoke up. Expressing his appreciation, he acknowledged the spiritual unity that had made this miracle possible: Noor was initially assessed by a Sikh doctor, the rescue process was carried out by a Christian nurse, and lastly, his daughter was freed from the pain by a Hindu engineering technician. Overwhelmed by this pure act of devotion, he also gave Santosh a token of gratitude, and said he would always be indebted to the Apollo team.

Story 8

Clothed in Kindness

Apollo BGS Hospitals, Mysuru

SIX-YEAR-OLD POONAM WAS BROUGHT TO APOLLO BGS Hospitals, Mysuru with severe burn injuries. While feeding her three-month-old brother, Poonam's mother had left boiling porridge on the stove. It had spilled on Poonam while she was romping around in the kitchen. She was rushed to the hospital and was diagnosed with 25 per cent burns. The disastrous incident left the little girl and her family traumatized.

After a series of surgeries, she was shifted to the ward to help her recover and start with slight movements. Since the burns were still raw, Poonam could not wear any clothes—she was only covered with dressings. This was a challenging time for the child, her parents as well as the attending staff, as Poonam refused to move out of her bed in this state. Her discomfort caught the attention of Sister Carunya, the assistant nursing superintendent. She designed four custom-tailored gowns made of gauze with the help of an in-house tailor, Mahadevaiah, for Poonam.

Since Poonam's condition was still very delicate, to prevent the spreading of any infection, the gowns were sent for autoclaving before they were put on her. Poonam agreed to wear the gown and started some mobility activities, and the dedication of Carunya and Mahadevaiah was finally fruitful. Within a few days, she began recovering and was finally discharged.

During her follow-up visits for skin toning and patching of the burnt areas, her parents never once failed to express their gratitude to Dr Narayan Hegde, the plastic surgeon, and other staff members for going out of their way to stitch those gowns for Poonam and for helping her recover both mentally and physically within a short duration. These small deeds boost the enthusiasm of Apollo's team and extend empathy to the patients in every possible way.

Story 9

Lost No Longer

Apollo BGS Hospitals, Mysuru

PRIYADARSHINI, A RESIDENT OF THE SMALL TOWN OF Talakkadu, was brought to Apollo BGS Hospitals, Mysuru in 2021 for the diagnosis and treatment of critical bleeding. Gynaecologist Dr Vanitha analysed her condition and performed a uterus removal surgery. Priyadarshini was accompanied by her younger son. Having spent all her life in her village and on farms, city life was a new and somewhat intimidating experience for her.

During her recovery at the hospital, Ms Jennifa Joy, senior executive of operations, became good friends with her. On her daily rounds, she interacted with Priyadarshini and asked her about her family, sons, and her life at the farm. On the day of Priyadarshini's discharge, Ms Jennifa asked her how she would be commuting back when released so that she could arrange for an ambulance, if required. That's when Priyadarshini opened up and said that she had to travel to Bengaluru to her elder son but had no idea how to reach there.

Seeing the anxiety and confusion in Priyadarshini's eyes, Ms Jennifa decided to help her. She approached Geeta, another staff member, and together, they made all the arrangements for Priyadarshini and her younger son. They booked the train tickets, escorted them to the station, and ensured that they were seated comfortably on their seats. They even coordinated with the elder son, informing him about the departure and arrival time of the train, so that he could be at the station to receive his mother and brother.

This kind deed left Priyadarshini speechless. Blessing Ms Jennifa from the heart, she, along with her sons, thanked the staff. Priyadarshini is still in contact with Ms Jennifa. She is doing well now, back at Talakkadu, and has also invited Ms Jennifa to her house whenever she visits that side.

Story 10

Mother's Touch

Apollo BGS Hospitals, Mysuru

NOT ONLY CARING FOR THE PATIENT BUT CARING FOR THEIR family is also equally important because recovery is as much a function of the mind as it is of physical healing. This was well-demonstrated by the Apollo BGS Hospitals, Mysuru staff when thirty-four-year-old Mayuri was brought to the emergency ward in 2021. She had suddenly collapsed in the wee hours of the morning, and Dr Somnath Vasudev had advised her to be admitted for observation.

During her daily rounds, Ms Motcharackini, deluxe ward in-charge, met Mayuri and realized that the lady was a bundle of nerves. She couldn't stop worrying about her five-month-old, whom she had left at home. Despite consolation from the nurse, Mayuri was terribly anxious and kept saying that she wanted to feed her baby. Considering this to be a delicate situation, the staff discussed it with Dr Somnath and took the necessary permissions from all other departments to get the baby to the hospital for feeding.

This was a critical decision because COVID was at its peak at the time, and all the other family members of Mayuri were down with viral fever. Though their RT-PCR reports were negative, the staff took extra precautions in getting the baby to her mother at the hospital.

Mayuri was dumbstruck when she saw the sister walking in with her baby. No words could have explained the hurricane of emotions she felt when holding her little one in her arms. The hungry baby began feeding at once, and both mother and child were happy.

Mayuri was kept under observation for three days, and the Apollo staff dutifully brought the baby every morning and safely dropped her back in the evening. Mayuri was highly appreciative of this extra care and thanked the staff for uniting them. Even today, when she visits the hospital for routine check-ups and gets the vaccinations for her baby from Paediatrician Dr Girish, she never fails to stop by to say hello to the deluxe ward staff, the service excellence team and the other staff members.

Story 11

A Gem of an Act

Apollo Speciality Hospitals, Madurai

ADMITTED TO THE STROKE UNIT IN MARCH 2022 AT APOLLO, Madurai, Madhavan, an eighty-four-year-old man, was struggling to stay alive. He had been diagnosed with subdural haematoma, a type of bleeding inside the head which occurs within the skull but is outside the actual brain tissue. Not only was his condition critical, but his wife, who accompanied him to the hospital, had also gone numb.

The bond between Madhavan and his wife was clearly visible. She wanted to save her husband and do the best for him, but the lack of financial resources was a big stumbling block. They hailed from a nearby village and were not even carrying any cash. Their only son was working in Chennai as a supervisor in a hotel and was unable to reach the hospital in time. Madhavan's wife was expressing her helplessness to one of her relatives on the phone when one of the hospital's nursing staff members, Bhuvana, heard the conversation. The old lady was offering to give away her golden studs in return for some financial help. The studs had been gifted to her by Madhavan on her birthday and were very close to her heart. But at this time, no precious jewellery was more important than her husband's life.

To soothe her anxious mind, Bhuvana asked her about the design of the golden studs and reassured her that everything would be fine. She shared the situation with the guest relations staff, and they decided to spring a happy surprise for the couple. The next morning, a mini gift was placed in her hands. She unwrapped the box and was astonished to see a pair of one-gram gold earrings similar to hers. She was speechless with emotion.

After a long period of anxiety, Madhavan was able to witness the joy on his wife's face, and the moment was priceless! He was discharged soon after and is doing well now, with only minimal support. Though his visit to Apollo, Madurai was short, the gesture of the hospital's staff will hold a special corner in the elderly couple's hearts forever.

Story 12

The Gift of a Smile

Apollo Hospitals, Nashik

THE EMERGENCY WARD STAFF WAS SHOCKED IN JULY 2022, when a five-year-old boy named Somesh Nayak was brought to Apollo Hospitals, Nashik. Though they would attend to severe casualties every day, this case was particularly unnerving. The boy had been mauled by a leopard while he was playing in his courtyard. His face, arms and legs had suffered multiple injuries.

While Somesh was physically injured, his parents had mentally collapsed. Somesh was their only son; his father was a simple farmer. It was a difficult sight for them to see their little boy suffer in agony.

General Surgeon Dr Milind Shah took the critical case into his experienced hands. With the treatment and medication, Somesh could not feel the pain, but the trauma had had an impact on his brain. The little boy was unconscious. It seemed like he did not want to gain consciousness, perhaps because the scene of the leopard attacking him was playing on repeat mode in his head.

Rashmi and Yamini, the staff in charge of counselling patients and their relatives, decided to do something special for Somesh. They decorated his room with posters of his favourite cartoons and balloons. When the boy finally opened his eyes, he was surprised to see the beautiful, colourful surroundings. His parents were relieved to see a hint of a smile on their child's face.

The efforts of the staff did not stop there. Throughout Somesh's recovery, they playfully interacted with the boy, bought him a magic slate, studied the alphabet with him, and played his favourite cartoon for him on television. This little effort by the Apollo team left a lasting imprint on the parents' hearts. They thanked the staff multiple times and even now after his discharge, when Somesh comes for check-ups, his parents never fail to express their gratitude for the staff and their thoughtful gestures.

Story 13

A Surprise Celebration

Apollo Hospitals, Nashik

SONALI'S HUSBAND DHEERAJ WAS ADMITTED TO APOLLO Hospitals, Nashik in June 2022 for total hip replacement under Orthopaedic Surgeon Dr Anil Jadhav. This was the same month when the 'Vat Purnima' festival is observed. This festival is celebrated by married women for three days every year in the north-western part of India. Women observe fasting and tie threads around a banyan tree, seeking their husbands' long and healthy lives as a blessing.

Sonali, a devoted wife, celebrated the festival every year without fail. But this year, she was in a dilemma as to whether to stay beside Dheeraj at the hospital or go home for the festival. While she wanted to perform the pooja, she did not want to leave her spouse alone in the hospital in the name of customary rituals.

Ms Rashmi, on learning about Sonali's problem, contacted Guest Relations Head Yamini. Together, they decided to help Sonali perform the rituals while by her husband's side. The staff sourced a branch from the banyan tree carefully planted in a pot and other items required for the ritual like flowers, bangles, sindoor, etc. During the peak hour of the pooja, the staff went to Sonali with all the preparations and asked her to perform the 'Vat Purnima'.

It was a complete surprise for Sonali, who was so touched that she burst into tears. The staff comforted her, and she performed all the rituals faithfully and peacefully. Not only Sonali, but also other relatives who had come to visit Dheeraj participated in the ceremony. It was a day to be remembered for a lifetime, both for Sonali and for the Apollo staff.

Dheeraj's surgery was successful, and he wholeheartedly thanked the entire staff. Sonali and Dheeraj never fail to express their gratitude even now when they visit Apollo for their routine follow-ups.

Story 14

The Spirit of Friendship

Apollo Hospitals, Nashik

LIFE WAS A LITTLE HARSH ON A HAPPY AND CHEERFUL LITTLE boy, Siddharth. Diagnosed with thalassemia and acute kidney injury, he was under the treatment of Dr Mohan Patel at Apollo Hospitals, Nashik. The only cure for this disease was a stem or bone marrow transplant; but both these procedures involved high risk and were only rarely recommended.

In Siddharth's case, doctors had advised his parents to just have faith in God and give their son as much happiness as possible. During one of his check-ups, Dr Mohan suggested admitting him for a few days and keeping him under observation.

Siddharth's condition did not allow him to live life like other normal boys. He could not walk and was bound to a wheelchair or his mother's lap for any type of movement. He did not even go to school and spent all his time at home. Despite his condition, Siddharth's enthusiasm never seemed to fade. But now, in the hospital, he had nothing much to do other than talk to his mother or stare at the monitoring screens. While on her routine rounds, one of the nurses, Rashmi, had a conversation with his mother about the boy's gloomy state; his mother said that he was miserable and missing his friends. She also told Rashmi that Siddharth loved playing carrom with his friends. This information was enough to ignite the passion in Apollo's staff of going the extra mile to care for the patients.

Quickly, with the help of Siddharth's mother, all his friends were brought to the hospital. All of them stayed some sixty kilometres from Nashik and their pick-up and drop were also arranged. A special set-up was done in the hospital's auditorium and Siddharth was brought there, unaware of the surprise that awaited him.

When he entered the auditorium, he squealed with joy to see all his friends. Dr Mohan himself was there, too. They played carrom and enjoyed snacks. The little act of kindness brought infinite happiness to Siddharth and his family.

Story 15

We'll Be Your Eyes

Apollo Hospitals, Nashik

DEPRIVED OF THE BEAUTY OF LIGHT AND COLOURS, VIPUL and his wife only had 10–15 per cent vision. Though they had adapted to their condition, it was challenging for them to navigate their way around new places. Thus, when they arrived at Apollo Hospitals, Nashik for a routine procedure under Dr Sheetal Gupta in August 2021, the nursing staff immediately noticed their discomfort in getting around.

In a snap of seconds, special arrangements were made for the couple.

The doctor advised Vipul to stay at the hospital for further observation. Rashmi, Yamini and the other nursing staff ensured that they were compassionately cared for and felt at home. A dedicated nurse was assigned to them, beds were allocated in proximity to the washrooms, and while the treatment progressed for Vipul, a guest relations associate kept his wife engaged, tending to her specific needs. On the day of discharge, the couple was escorted back home by a team of nurses in a fully equipped vehicle to ensure that they did not face any problems.

Well, the dedication of the Apollo staff to do that extra bit does not end here! Even after discharge, when the couple called customer care informing them that they could not visit the hospital for the routine follow-up, the hospital staff decided that if the patient cannot visit the hospital, the hospital should go to the patient.

Rashmi and Yamini, along with the ER team and the ambulance team, arranged for a pick-up vehicle to be sent for Vipul and his wife. They were brought to the hospital and the entire process of getting the blood tests was done, and the routine check-up was expedited. The reports were arranged on an emergency basis, and the team made sure that the entire process was finished on the same day. Later, the hospital team even dropped the couple back home.

During this entire course of treatment, Vipul and his wife truly admired the compassionate care that the hospital offered. They acknowledged that Apollo had changed their view of hospitals as being only profit-making organizations. 'Apollo Hospital and its staff will always have a special respect and remembrance in our hearts,' said Vipul.

Story 16

Together in Testing Times

Apollo Hospitals, Nashik

ABHISHEK, A CLASS X STUDENT, WAS RETURNING FROM THE examination centre after his penultimate board paper when he met with an unfortunate accident. His left leg was badly injured, and he was wheeled into the emergency ward of Apollo Hospitals, Nashik in April 2022. Dr Anil, the orthopaedic surgeon, concluded that he needed immediate surgery.

This was devastating news for the family. The surgery, though unavoidable, could crush Abhishek's dream of clearing his board examinations. If he missed the last paper, he would have to repeat class X, which in turn would set him back by a whole year in his career plans.

Of course, the Apollo staff could not let this happen. While Abhishek's operation day was yet to be decided and the boy was shifted to the ward, Yamini and Rashmi consulted Dr Jadhav and asked if he could somehow appear for the examination. The doctor, though compassionate about his situation, had to say no. He explained that Abhishek would have to undergo critical surgery, after which it would be impossible for the boy to move, let alone go to the examination hall and attempt the exam.

However, the staff did not give up. Four days after the surgery, they approached Dr Jadhav again. This time he gave permission, but with strict instructions to not overexert the boy and ensure that he did not move from the stretcher. Though it was only half the battle won, Rashmi, Nikhil and Siva Reddy joined the boy's school in seeking consent from the Nashik Board authorities to allow Abhishek to appear for the examination, accompanied in an ambulance by a scribe and a nursing staff member.

Taking extra precautions and safety measures, Abhishek was transferred to the examination centre in an ambulance with a resident doctor and nursing staff's aid, administered by Dr Mitesh Nikam, the AMS, and Libin, the nursing head, and with the assistance of a scribe, Abhishek attempted the exam.

The day Abhishek's result was announced, he and his father especially came to the hospital to share the news that Abhishek had cleared the board exams with 60 per cent marks. They wholeheartedly thanked the entire staff, without whose help this would not have been possible. Six months after the incident, Abhishek is back to walking normally and studying in class XI.

Story 17

Finding His Voice Again

Apollo Hospitals, Nashik

'MUSIC IS A THERAPY. IT IS A COMMUNICATION, FAR MORE powerful than words, far more immediate and sometimes even far more efficient than medicine.' This quote was rightly proven in the case of Arun Waghmare, a professor by occupation and a singer by heart.

Arun suddenly fell unconscious at home and was admitted to Apollo Hospitals, Nashik in July 2022 under the supervision of Dr Sanjay Vekhande. An emergency craniotomy surgery was performed on him. It is a critical brain surgery that involves removing part of the skull to access the brain. The skull bone is replaced when the surgery is done.

Though the surgery was a success, it limited his ability to speak. Even two to three days after the surgery, not a single whisper left his throat. The doctor recommended speech therapy for Arun, but the therapists found most of their efforts to be in vain.

While taking her daily rounds, Rashmi struck up a conversation with Arun's wife, and learnt that Arun was a very good singer and passionate about music. This gave her an idea. She spoke to Resident Medical Officer Dr Jaya, and they began making arrangements to get back Arun's lost voice. With the help of his wife, Arun's close friends were invited and a set-up with karaoke was prepared to surprise Arun at the CME hall.

Nurse Superintendent Libin, a good singer himself, also joined the gala event along with Dr Sanjay. When Arun was escorted to the hall, he was stunned to see all the preparations done especially for him. When Libin started singing and took the mic to Arun, his voice initially quivered. But soon, he was singing! Delighted, his wife began to dance.

Everyone enjoyed the moment. What speech therapy could not achieve, musical therapy had made possible! Arun recently underwent cranioplasty surgery, a procedure required after the craniotomy surgery. He is now back home and leading a normal life, mesmerizing his friends and family with his sweet voice.

Story 18

A Little Bundle of Joy

Apollo Hospitals, Bhubaneswar

BEING A MOTHER IS THE WORLD'S BEST FEELING, AND WHEN you hold the little one for the first time in your arms, the emotions cannot be explained in words. However, Damyanti had been deprived of this joy even after nine years of marriage. A happy homemaker and an entrepreneur, she desperately longed for a child.

Finally, she conceived a baby through the in vitro fertilization (IVF) procedure. But her joy turned to shock when a triple marker test in the sixth month revealed that the foetus had anorectal malformation. Even though Dr Sahu, her gynaecologist, comforted her that the condition was treatable and that the baby would be normal, she was inconsolable.

Soon after her delivery in April 2022, it was discovered that the baby boy had a problem with his legs at birth. Not only that, but he was also passing stool through the urethra instead of the rectum. The baby was immediately put under the care of Paediatric Surgeon Dr Antaryami. A sigmoid colostomy was performed on him, and it was a difficult time for the parents.

Despite all the complications, the little one turned out to be a fighter. He survived all the surgeries and medical procedures. After the surgery, when Damyanti held and fed her little bundle of joy, it was the moment of a lifetime for her. Steadily, the baby started to take up feed and was discharged in April 2022.

Damyanti and her baby are doing well now, and whenever the duo visit for follow-ups, they never fail to thank the entire Apollo team for their expert help and support.

Story 19

Mother and Child

Apollo Hospitals, Bannerghatta, Bengaluru

SURMANI AND HER HUSBAND HAD BECOME PARENTS AFTER many years of marriage. Their baby was just three months old when Surmani started experiencing some neurological issues. The couple came to Apollo Hospitals, Bannerghatta in March 2022 to visit Neurologist Dr Guru Charan, who advised that Surmani be admitted for treatment.

Even though the neurotherapy was essential, the couple were terribly anxious about their infant. While they were discussing what to do, GRE Head Ms Gitanjali overheard them and assured them that the hospital would do its best to take care of their baby.

The couple were told that the staff at Apollo Hospital were well-equipped and well-trained to take care of newborn babies. Ms Gitanjali briefed them about all the facilities and informed them that paediatricians were available on call round the clock. This was very comforting for Surmani and her husband.

The staff arranged for a private room near the neonatal ward. Sister Sujata, the nurse-in-charge of the neonatal ward, delegated duties of the baby to the best of her team. Starting from feeding the baby, to bathing and dressing, the nurses catered to every single need of the little one, by rotation.

After six days, when Surmani was discharged, the couple were amazed to see the dedication of the staff and thanked them a million times for this gesture. They even regretted not having had the delivery at Apollo but pledged to keep Apollo as their single destination in future for any medical requirement.

Story 20

Friends in Need

Apollo Hospitals, Ramnagar, Visakhapatnam

SUFFERING FROM CHRONIC KIDNEY DISEASE (CKD) AND LIVER cirrhosis, Prabhakar Sen had given up hope and was counting the days before his departure from the world. His family, out of spirits and also out of funds, brought him to Apollo Hospitals, Ramnagar as their last hope.

During his stay at the hospital, Prabhakar was really depressed and kept saying, 'Nothing is going to help me heal, let me just go home. I cannot afford the treatment. I have no money left.'

Dr Anusha, along with nursing staff members Lakshami and Shanti Priya, counselled him to be optimistic. They also apprised Deputy Medical Superintendent Prasad of the couple's financial situation. He took matters into his hands, and with the help of Prabhakar's wife, personally called upon his relatives to provide them with financial aid. His efforts bore results and 70 per cent of the billing amount was raised and the remaining 30 per cent was generously waived by the hospital.

With the cumulative efforts of his family members, doctors, nursing staff, and Prasad, Prabhakar's treatment was successful. On the day of his discharge, Prabhakar ordered sweets for the entire staff as a small token of love and appreciation, and the couple even clicked photographs with the staff, while thanking them from the heart.

Story 21

Her Last Blessing

Apollo Speciality Hospital, Jayanagar, Bengaluru

In July 2021, Priya was scouring the Internet for a suitable bride for her youngest son, when she suddenly felt breathless and was rushed to Apollo Speciality Hospital, Jayanagar, Bengaluru. She was immediately shifted to the isolation ward and put on a ventilator. In view of her deteriorating condition, Dr Ravindra Mehta recommended dialysis.

Throughout the treatment, Priya was worried about her son's marriage, because her instinct told her she did not have long to live. Over the next few days, she was also diagnosed with cancer. Her chemotherapy sessions began, but the doctors knew that her survival chances were minimal.

Knowing how much her son meant to her, her family members expedited the search for a bride. Fortunately, a suitable match was found, and wedding arrangements were made at the earliest, with only minimal preparations and guests.

When the intensive care unit (ICU) team, consisting of Dr Madhusudhan and one of the allocation staff members, Pushpa, learnt about Priya's last wish, they contacted the information technology (IT) team and made all the necessary arrangements for Priya to witness the wedding proceedings from her bed in the ICU in the early hours.

The next day, the newlywed couple visited Priya to seek her blessings, and it was like Priya was holding her last breath only for this day. She peacefully passed away the following day.

Priya began her next journey, but her memories and the kind deeds of the Apollo team will always have a special place in her family members' hearts.

Story 22

A Gift of Solace

Apollo Children's Hospital, Chennai

RUKMANI'S NINETEEN-DAY-OLD BABY WAS ADMITTED TO Apollo Children's Hospital, Chennai under the Chief Minister Scheme (CMS) in February 2022 under the guidance of Primary Consultant Dr C.S. Muthukumaran. The family came from a very poor background, and were visiting all the way from Kumbakonam. However, they did not want to leave any stone unturned to seek the best treatment for their baby.

Rukmani's baby was referred for congenital cardiac heart surgery under Cardiothoracic Surgeon Dr Neville Solomon. On the same day as the admission, the surgery was conducted, but the baby could not make it through and bid adieu to the world in the same month. The parents were devastated.

Though the bills were cleared from the CMS fund, because of their financial incapability, the parents did not even have enough money left to take the deceased body back home. They approached the chief security officer, Mr Suresh, and the unit head, Mrs Niranjani S. Mr Suresh was apprised of the situation. He arranged for an ambulance at the minimal cost of Rs 3,000 for the baby to be taken back home. But the parents did not have even this much money. In fact, they were not even sure how they would perform the last rites of the baby.

Seeing their heart-wrenching situation, Mr Suresh approached the other departments and requested them to raise money for the little one. Many of the staff members from the billing and administration departments, including Mr Sakthi and Mr Nanda, ward secretary members, including Mr Kesavan and Ms Chellammal, insurance desk staff members, including Ms Surya Kala and other nursing staff members, together managed to collect a handsome amount.

The raised money was handed over to Rukmani and her husband, and the deputy general manager ordered that the ambulance and the driver be paid for from the hospital's petty cash. Even though Rukmani's baby could not survive, these small and unselfish efforts of the Apollo team ensured that both the parents and the baby found peace.

Story 23

Reading as Therapy

Apollo Adlux, Kochi

JUST TWENTY-EIGHT YEARS OLD, JOSENA MET WITH AN accident in August 2021 and was admitted to Apollo Adlux, Kochi. The terrifying incident left her in shock, and she withdrew into a shell. Day after day passed, but the girl refused to even speak to anyone.

While her primary treatment was going on, Psychiatrist Dr Anu started counselling her, trying to get her to open up. Initially, the sessions did not bring in any positive results. However, after a few days, when Dr Anu became more familiar with Josena, she suggested reading therapy. She herself picked a few selected books from her therapeutic collection at home and brought them to her. Next, she asked Josena's attendant and brother, Bipin, to read a few selected portions from those books to her on a regular basis.

Gradually, Josena started responding to the reading sessions and started opening up. She was able to share the horrific memories of the incident with her near and dear ones. Seeing their daughter finally break out of the burdening cage of the horrific accident, her parents were greatly relieved. Slowly, Josena returned to her normal self and was discharged a month later.

Her parents wholeheartedly thanked Dr Anu, Brother Bipin and all the Apollo staff members for taking care of their daughter and offering the reading therapy treatment, which had been immensely successful. When Josena and her parents left the hospital, their happy faces made the hospital staff smile.

Story 24

A Timely Touch

Apollo Adlux, Kochi

IN SEPTEMBER 2021, WHEN SIXTY-THREE-YEAR-OLD Chandraswami left home for his evening walk, he had no idea he would land up in hospital. But he suffered a sudden cardiac arrest, and was rushed to Apollo Adlux, Kochi in an unconscious state. Fortunately, the incident happened close to the hospital.

It seemed like luck was on Chandraswami's side. Just when he fell to the ground, security guard Binoy was returning home after completing his night shift. As soon as Binoy spotted Chandraswami, he rushed forward to help. He realized that the man's pulse was very feeble and that his blood pressure seemed to be dropping rapidly. Without panicking, he called the ambulance and took the old man to the hospital.

Chandraswami was treated at the emergency ward and was later shifted to the ICU. Meanwhile, Binoy checked his last-dialled calls and got in touch with his family members.

Under the timely ministration of Dr Jay Krishnan, it was discovered that Chandraswami had 100 per cent blockage in his heart and required immediate action. An angioplasty was conducted the same day, and Chandraswami's life was saved.

While recovering at the hospital, Chandraswami also established a bond with Nurse Aparna, who gifted him a ceramic mug on his departure two weeks later. Even now, when Chandraswami visits the hospital for follow-ups, he makes sure that he does not leave the hospital without asking about Binoy and extending his gratitude to the staff.

Story 25

Reconnected

Apollo Hospitals, Tondiarpet

A devoted son, sixty-seven-year-old Jacob never married so that he could look after his beloved mother. After her demise, he had become quite lonely. However, he had forged deep bonds with the staff at Apollo Hospitals, Tondiarpet. He had been coming to the hospital for twenty years for every medical need, big or small. So much so that whenever he faced a medical emergency, a room would be pre-booked for him with all the arrangements made in advance.

But one day, he was wheeled into the hospital in an unconscious state. Dr Kannayan diagnosed him with severe breathing difficulty and severe back ache, for which he was put under treatment. When he came around, he told the staff that he had broken his phone and had no way of communicating with anyone.

Unit Head Mr Bhavani Shekhar, who was quite close to the old man, gifted him a brand-new phone. The staff also assured him that Apollo was just a call away whenever he needed them. To make him feel comfortable and always at home, special meals consisting of his favourite dishes were provided to him throughout his stay at the hospital.

Touched by the surprise gifts and the kindness extended to him, Jacob wholeheartedly thanked Bhavani and the other staff members and said that he was blessed to have a family at Apollo.

Story 26

An Angel to the Rescue

Apollo Adlux, Kochi

THE DATE WAS 23 APRIL 2022. SHEEBA, A NEURO NURSING staff member at Apollo Adlux, Kochi was travelling back home in a moderately crowded bus after her shift. Everything seemed just normal like every day when she suddenly felt a touch from behind. She looked back, only to see a young man falling from his seat.

Sheeba rushed to his help and checked his pulse. There was none. She decided to give him cardiopulmonary resuscitation (CPR), and while struggling to revive him, requested the passengers to help. Nobody came forward. She was disheartened but pulled the young man towards the footboard and gave him a second cycle of CPR. Even with the second round, the man did not regain his pulse. From the symptoms, it seemed to be a clear case of epilepsy.

Sheeba turned the man on his stomach and started rubbing his back vigorously. At last, the man gained consciousness and was rushed to the nearest hospital.

Sheeba's spontaneous act of bravery not only saved the man's life, but also made the Apollo family proud of having her as a member of the team. Appreciation poured in to salute her for her prompt action. She was also honoured in the presence of the MP and MLA of the constituency.

Story 27

A Real-Life Hero

Apollo Adlux, Kochi

It was Alvin's first day of work at Apollo Adlux, Kochi in December 2021. He had no idea that he would be performing a heroic act on that very day.

That day, a patient named Mr Kumaran was being discharged to go home. He had been brought to the hospital with severe injuries from an accident and had now recovered sufficiently to be put under home care.

While Mr Kumaran's discharge formalities were underway, his stretcher was parked in the lobby, ready to be taken to the ambulance. The stretcher rested on a trolley, and an attendant stood beside it. He had left the trolley for just a few moments, to take last minute instructions from the doctor. And that is when something dangerous happened.

The trolley malfunctioned and began to skid. The patient lost his balance and started falling. Just then, Alvin took on the scene and rushed to stop the trolley. He swiftly saved the patient from any further injuries than he was already suffering from his first accident. Things changed from normal to adverse and back to ordinary in a blink of an eye.

Even before anyone could think or understand what had just happened, an about-to-happen misfortune was bravely avoided by Alvin's spontaneous response. However, he himself suffered a shoulder dislocation. He was offered free treatment from the hospital and received a reward from Mr Kumaran's family. Apollo authorities also commended his heroic effort.

Story 28

Six Swift Gifts

Apollo Adlux, Kochi

In November 2021, Philip's son, admitted to Apollo Adlux, Kochi was declared brain dead. The tragedy hit Philip hard and left him depressed.

Once he came to terms with his loss, however, the bereaved father realized that though nothing could bring his son back, he could still keep him alive through different people. Philip expressed his wish to donate his son's organs. This was the first organ donation at Apollo Adlux, Kochi from a patient.

As soon as Philip's wish was conveyed to the higher management, immediate arrangements were made, and the responsible authorities made greater efforts in furnishing the organs to the seeking recipients across the state. In no time, suitable beneficiaries were found, and the organs were able to resurrect six lives. While the body of the deceased was taken for his last rituals, his soul remained alive through six different people.

Just a few days later this courageous act, Nation Organ Donation Day was observed on 27 November 2021. On this occasion, the management of Apollo Adlux invited Philip, acknowledging his generous deed, and saluted him and his family for the noble gesture. A frame of souvenirs was given to Philip to memorialize his departed son; and it was also the hospital's way of showing a token of gratitude. In this instance, the hospital became a means of standing by a noble cause.

Story 29

Lost and Found

Apollo Women's Hospital, Chennai

Ashima Ghosh came to Apollo Women's Hospital, Chennai for a routine check-up in January 2022. Her husband, Subhash, accompanied her. Dr Sumana Manohar examined Ashima and told her that everything was normal. The couple left the hospital, only to return a few hours later, in a state of anxiety.

Upon enquiry, Subhash said that his wife's purse was missing, and it had quite a few important documents and valuable items. Duty Security Supervisor Ashok was approached for the matter, and he in turn informed Chief Security Officer Suresh Kumar.

The team launched a search for the missing purse. CCTV footage of the associated areas where the couple had been revealed that Ashima was still holding the purse when they had left the hospital premises. Even so, Mr Kumar assisted the couple in finding it. His team went to the nearby auto stand, from where the couple had boarded a rickshaw. The rickshaw driver denied finding any purse in his vehicle. Kumar then took the couple to the clothing store where Ashima and Subhash had gone to shop. The missing purse was found at the store. After checking for all the documents and valuables, they thanked the store owner and left.

While the team breathed a sigh of relief, Ashima and Subhash expressed their gratitude to the entire security team of Apollo for helping them locate the purse.

Story 30

A Dramatic Rescue

Apollo Speciality Hospitals, Vanagaram

In March 2022, a lady, crying bitterly, walked into Apollo Hospital, Vanagaram with the sub-inspector of police. Her seven-year-old daughter had gone missing, and during the investigation, it had been revealed that the kidnapper might be someone belonging to West Bengal. The CCTV footage of the area from where the child had been picked up showed that a woman with north-eastern facial features had abducted the kid.

The police had also been tipped off that the kidnapper might be lurking somewhere in the vicinity of the hospital. That is why they had gone there, hoping to get some information from a staff member or a probe into the migrant staff list.

The inspector approached Head of Security Mr Nasardeen and checked with the security team as well but found no clue. Further, the case was taken up to housekeeping and the food and beverage department as there were north-eastern staff members working in these departments. At first, he approached Head of the Department of Housekeeping Mr Sivakumar. He came upfront to help with who all he had seen at the entrance, and he assured the inspector of CCTV footage through Mr Nasardeen, who also in turn assured his team's full cooperation. The image of the kidnapped girl, extracted from the video footage, was circulated among the staff members. But nobody had any information.

With no hope of seeing her daughter again, the mother broke down. Just before the police left the hospital, they were informed that Dhanush, an old employee of the hospital, had left for the night after his duty. The authorities felt he might know something about the suspect, since he had been a part of the Apollo family for over a decade and had been a senior staff member in the housekeeping team for more than three years.

Dhanush was summoned to the hospital. As soon as he saw the footage of the lady, he recognized her. She was a migrant worker, and he had interacted with her community quite often. The police team hurried to the location with Dhanush and apprehended the suspect.

It was a touching moment when the girl flew into her mother's arms. While everyone celebrated the reunion, Dhanush was highly appreciated for his prompt and heroic task in helping the police catch the accused. The local police commissioner personally called Dhanush for extending his help and rewarded him. The hospital management also awarded him a letter of appreciation.

Story 31

The Angel Next Door

Apollo Speciality Hospitals, Vanagaram

IT WAS A DARK AND STORMY NIGHT. JOSEPH WAS DRIVING IN the blinding rain, trying to get his wife Maria to the hospital in time. Their situation was critical. Maria had previously suffered a newborn's death and a miscarriage and was now in labour again.

The couple almost gave up hope when the car broke down. It seemed like destiny had planned a rather dramatic entry for the baby.

Suddenly, Joseph remembered that a nurse lived in the vicinity. Luckily, Ms Antoniammal, a midwife from Apollo Hospital, Vanagaram, was in her hometown to spend her annual holidays with her mother. From the moment he knocked on her door, Antoniammal took charge of the situation. She quickly examined Maria and saw that the baby's head was fully engaged. And as if the complications were not enough, there was a complete blackout in the village due to the bad weather. Using a hurricane lamp, a pair of sterile scissors, and some courage, the nurse proceeded to conduct the delivery.

It was complicated. The umbilical cord was coiled around the baby's neck and shoulder. She skilfully released it and manoeuvred the baby out. The healthy baby boy let out a strong wail, lighting up his parents' hearts. Using the controlled cord traction method, she completely separated the placenta and cleaned up both mother and child.

Back at the hospital, Antoniammal received huge appreciation for her generous act of kindness. She was also honoured with multiple awards, including the Service Excellence Award and a Letter of Excellence in the presence of the IP head and heads of departments, along with JDMS Dr Paul and COO and DMS of Cluster 2, Dr Rahul.

Story 32

Helping Hands

Apollo Speciality Hospitals, Vanagaram

ACCOMPANIED BY HER DAUGHTER, MEERA NAIR WAS admitted to Apollo Hospital, Vanagaram for multiple medical conditions, under the care of General Physician Dr M.D. Selvam and the neurology department. She was soon to be discharged.

While on one hand, the mother and daughter were happy to go home, they were quite worried as to how they would cope with Meera's fragile health. The lady was too weak even to walk up to the lift.

When Head of the Department of Facility Management Services Mr Sivakumar learnt of their predicament, he assured them that all the patients at Apollo are treated as family members, and that they would receive full support on transportation and assistance. True to his word, Mr Sivakumar arranged for a vehicle and two staff members, Akila and Milan, to accompany the mother and daughter and make sure that they reach home safe and sound. Akila and Milan not only took them home, but also cleaned up the house and set their luggage in place.

Meera and her daughter had not expected the hospital to extend this much help. They expressed their sincere gratitude to the Apollo staff, and even today, when they visit for follow-ups, they never fail to leave the premises without calling Mr Sivakumar and thanking him for his generosity.

Story 33

The Lunchbox

Apollo Reach Hospital, Karaikudi

MADHUSUDAN WAS A REGULAR VISITOR OF APOLLO REACH Hospital, Karaikudi. In November 2021, he came to the hospital for his periodic check-up, but that day his physician, Dr Saravana Kumar, had to attend to an emergency case. All the patients waiting for the doctor were apologized to for the delay and were requested to have lunch by the time the doctor would next be available.

Madhusudan had not eaten since morning because he expected to be back home by lunchtime. He had been advised not to eat outside food, so he just sat outside the out-patient department. The clock ticked, and by the time it was Madhusudan's turn to consult the doctor, it was already somewhere around 4 in the evening. When, finally, his investigation was over and he came out of the doctor's chamber, he was famished. It would take him two hours to reach home.

By now, his hunger was unbearable. He went to the hospital canteen and got himself a coffee, thinking something would be better than nothing. The elderly man's distressed condition caught the eye of housekeeping staff member Jesudoss, who brought it to the notice of the unit's food and beverage manager, Sridhar.

When Sridhar came to know that the old man was hungry since morning, he quickly went to his room and got his lunchbox. He generously offered his home-cooked food to Madhusudan. Deeply touched, Madhusudan declined, saying he did not want to deprive Sridhar of his food. But Sridhar reassured him, saying he would order something for himself.

A tear rolled out of Madhusudan's eye. In Sridhar, he saw his own son, whom he had lost a few months back in an accident. After having lunch, he left the hospital with a full stomach and respect in his heart for Sridhar's kind deed.

Story 34

In the Nick of Time

Apollo Reach Hospital, Karaikudi

IN DECEMBER 2021, APOLLO REACH HOSPITAL, KARAIKUDI housekeeping staff member Jesudoss was heading home after completing his night shift. On his way home, just a few miles away from the hospital, he spotted a man lying in a pool of blood. The man had been hit by a van and had suffered severe injuries.

Jesudoss rushed towards the man and sensed the seriousness of the situation. Without any delay, he called the emergency team and asked for an ambulance. Meanwhile, using basic life support techniques, he kept the man's pulse ticking. When the ambulance arrived, Jesudoss jumped in beside the patient, even though he had been awake all night.

As soon as the patient reached the hospital, a team took charge, and his admission process was expedited under the RTA. While Orthopaedist Dr Asai Selvan was examining the patient and attending to his injuries, one of the staff members of the admissions department, Rajkumar, took on the responsibility to track down the person's identity.

It was found and confirmed that the patient's name was Keshavnand, and his kids were immediately informed about the unfortunate incident. When the family hastily reached the hospital, Jesudoss was the first person to meet them. He assured them that Keshavnand was in good hands.

By now, the doctors had begun their treatment and were seeking blood for Keshavnand, who had a rare blood group. Once again, Jesudoss came to his rescue. His blood group matched that of Keshavnand, and he at once volunteered to donate blood. Despite a terrible spine injury, Keshavnand began to respond gradually, and Jesudoss remained alongside the patient all the while he was in the ICU. Within three days, the man was discharged from the hospital.

Before leaving, the patient and his family gave a million thanks to Jesudoss, who had saved Keshavnand's life. After the patient's departure from the hospital, much appreciation was showered on Jesudoss for his benevolence, and the entire Apollo Reach Hospital, Karaikudi family was proud of him.

Story 35

A Bond of Affection

Apollo Reach Hospital, Karaikudi

ESHVARDUTT AND HIS WIFE DEVANGANA WERE IN THEIR sunset years. They had no children and no family, except each other. With the passing years, Eshvardutt developed an ailment and was admitted to Apollo Reach Hospital, Karaikudi in December 2021 under the supervision of Dr Thirupathy Sankarlingam.

The treatment required the removal of Eshvardutt's leg. Besides the major surgery, what worried them was the expense involved. Even their life's entire savings were not enough for the treatment, and a bank loan seemed to be the only option. But the couple had no idea how to apply for a loan. They didn't even possess debit or credit cards.

That's when Learning and Development Coordinator Umayal volunteered to help them. Her husband worked in a bank, and she got him to explain basic banking procedure to the couple. With his help, they were issued a debit card on priority basis.

Due to some complications, Eshvardutt's stay was extended for a little longer. During his recovery, Devangana's bond with Umayal strengthened even more. Umayal got them home-cooked food daily and even brought them pongal on the day of the festival. Devangana saw the daughter she never had in Umayal. Their affinity towards each other grew stronger by the day.

On the day of Eshvardutt's discharge, the housekeeping team gifted the couple a towel origami—a small baby made out of towel, custom-made for them. The team's gesture touched the couple to the core, and they left the hospital beaming with joy.

Story 36

A Daughter's Dilemma

Apollo Reach Hospital, Karaikudi

FIFTY-SEVEN-YEAR-OLD AAISHA HAD BEEN A REGULAR visitor at Apollo Reach Hospital, Karaikudi for the past six years for her dialysis treatment under Dr Saravana Kumar. Generally, Aaisha's daughter accompanied her mother to the hospital. However, during one of her visits in 2021, she was unable to make it because her baby was unwell.

Aaisha was taken in for dialysis, but her daughter fretted outside the unit, debating whether to stay or to go home.

One of the hospital's dieticians, Ms Popsoaa, was on her daily rounds and happened to notice the daughter's distress. Upon learning of the problem, Popsoaa assured her that Aaisha would be taken care of with absolute attentiveness and asked her to go home and look after her baby.

After three hours, when Aaisha's dialysis was done, housekeeping staff member Pandimeenal assisted the lady. Without telling her what had happened, Pandimeenal just informed her that her daughter had to leave for some urgent work. Pandimeenal's care did not stop here; she went ahead and called her husband, an auto-rickshaw driver, to drop Aaisha safely at her home.

Without bothering about the payment of the fare, Pandimeenal's husband took Aaisha to her home with utmost safety. On seeing her mother entering, with all due care, assisted by Pandimeenal and her husband, Aaisha's daughter was greatly relieved. She thanked the staff for the extra help and for taking care of her mother while she was not there.

Story 37

Commendable Charity

Apollo Speciality Hospitals, Nellore

THINGS DID NOT GO AS EXPECTED FOR NARAYAN AND HIS wife when they visited Apollo Speciality Hospitals, Nellore, to consult Urologist Dr Nishchal Prasad. The couple had travelled from a remote native land all the way to Nellore, seeking treatment under Arogyasari, a dedicated insurance scheme by the government of Andhra Pradesh. However, they were shocked to learn that the scheme was no more operational at Apollo.

This information left the couple in distress, and they wondered how to afford the treatment. Ms Madhavi, one of the nurses in the urology department, noticed their sadness and brought it to the notice of Dr Nischal Prasad. Being a kind-hearted doctor, he sympathized with the couple and volunteered to help them out. He not only offered free consultation to Narayan, but also waived the entire treatment cost.

The couple was much obliged for this generous act and poured blessings of abundance and prosperity for Dr Nischal Prasad, Ms Madhavi and the Apollo staff. The extended care for Narayan and his wife did not stop there. Since it would be a long and tiring journey back home for the couple, Ms Madhavi also made arrangements from the hospital canteen and ensured that the couple did not leave on an empty stomach.

Emotional and tearful, the couple left the hospital with immense gratitude in their hearts.

Story 38

An Act of Empathy

Apollo Research Hospital, Indore

DINESH, A PATIENT OF DIABETES AND HYPERTENSION, suddenly started feeling breathless one day. The month was April 2022, and with every passing minute, his condition was deteriorating. His wife began to panic.

In the middle of the chaos, she remembered Usha, her next-door neighbour, and dialled her number. Usha had been a dedicated member of Apollo Hospital, Indore's staff for the past twelve years. Seeing Dinesh's wife's number flashing on her screen, Usha picked up the call instantly.

Hearing the quivering voice, Usha sensed that immediate action was required. She called the emergency unit, arranged for an ambulance to be sent to Dinesh's house, consulted Dr Pranay Bhaskar, the doctor-in-charge, and even made pre-arrangements to receive the patient and immediately start the treatment.

As soon as Dinesh was brought to the hospital, Dr Pranay began treatment. Dinesh was suffering from haemothorax. His blood platelets were fast decreasing. He was shifted to the ICU.

Dinesh's wife stood outside, fretting about how to pay the bills. Usha knew about their financial condition and volunteered to help. Along with other staff members and with the help of the church and hospital authorities, she managed to raise a handsome amount of Rs 2,00,000 for Dinesh.

Though Dinesh's condition improved, and he was discharged, he passed away some time after. However, his wife will always remain grateful to Usha and the other staff members for their timely and generous help.

Story 39

Art Therapy

Apollo Hospital, Karur

A HIGHLY TALENTED AND CREATIVE GIRL, CHANDNI, WAS brought to Apollo Hospital, Karur in January 2022. She had some symptoms of acute tropical ailment and was admitted under the supervision of General Physician Dr Senthil Muthu. It was diagnosed that Chandni was suffering from first-stage dengue. She was therefore admitted to the hospital.

However, as days passed, Chandni grew increasingly bored and despondent. During her daily rounds, Anita, a clinical dietician and also the person responsible for service excellence, noticed Chandni's wistful expression. She spoke to Chandni's mother and discovered that the girl was a talented artist and an art and craft teacher in a school. Her mother said that Chandni's artfully busy hands were missing their creative work, in turn sending her into depression.

Anita decided to cheer Chandni up. She, along with the other guest relations team members, arranged for Lippan art accessories like clay, mirrors, cloth, paint, etc. The next day, Chandni was delighted to find all these items next to her bedside, and beamed ear-to-ear after several days. In no time, her skilled hands were at work. Her body was gradually recovering from dengue, and her artful mind was now fruitfully occupied.

On the day of her discharge, Chandni offered a fine piece of Lippan art to Anita and the team as a gesture of thanks. To the staff, the smile in her eyes was ample reward for their efforts.

Story 40

Call of Duty

Apollo Proton Cancer Centre (APCC)

IT WAS PAST MIDNIGHT IN APRIL 2022, WHEN A LOUD telephone ring broke the silence of the otherwise quiet night at APCC. The screen was displaying a landline number and Dipak, the on-duty manager at APCC, received the call but could hear only a faint mumbling on the other side of the line. With much effort, he could manage to grasp only a few words like 'chest pain, Somerset Hotel, Room No 1008'. Before he could understand anything else or ask something, the call got disconnected. He sensed that it was an emergency call.

Dipak immediately called Somerset Hotel and inquired with the lobby manager to check on the occupant of room number 1008. Indeed, they found that the guest, Mr Saurabh Deskhmukh, was suffering from severe chest pain. An ambulance was rushed to the hotel, and since Apollo Spectra was the nearest hospital, the patient was taken there. The lobby manager called Dipak back and informed him of the development.

Without wasting a moment, Dipak got to work and discovered that Mr Deshmukh was an existing patient of APCC and regularly visited the hospital for his chemotherapy under Dr Sujith Kumar Mullapally. By the time emergency care was provided at Apollo Spectra, Dipak arranged for an ambulance to be sent to the hospital, to pick up the patient and shift him to APCC. He also informed Saurabh's family members about the emergency.

It was half past one when Saurabh was received at APCC with all the pre-arrangements made and the on-call doctor attended to the patient. After thorough surveillance, Saurabh was discharged on the following day itself. With Dipak's timely action, a priceless life was saved.

Story 41

Healing a Broken Heart

APCC

SEVENTY-FIVE-YEAR-OLD JAMES STOOD IN A CORNER, SPEAKING to his wife on the public phone. Between sobs, he told her that he would be coming home since he did not have a smartphone to complete the registration process. James was at APCC to collect his son's samples and had just received the devastating news that the cancer had advanced.

Fincy, a guest relations officer at the hospital, overheard his conversation. She waited for him to hang up, and then went up to him and offered him a bottle of water. She asked him to share his problems with her. James told her that COVID had drained his family of all resources, and he had been hungry since morning.

With words of comfort, Fincy consoled James. Then she took out her phone and completed the online registration for him. Following this, she took him to the canteen and ordered food for him.

James called his son with renewed hope. He told him that God had sent an angel their way. Fincy's generosity didn't end there. She even handed over some money to James for the cab he would be taking home. James was speechless and thanked the Lord for sending this divine soul for his help.

The very next day, the cancer victim's little daughter and wife personally visited APCC to extend their gratitude to Fincy in person on behalf of the patient.

Story 42

A Disaster Averted

Apollo Main Hospital, Greams Road, Chennai

FOR THREE FULL DAYS IN SEPTEMBER 2021, RAIN POUNDED on Chennai. Mahadevi, a seventy-two-year-old lady from Kolathur, was a regular patient at Apollo Main Hospital, Chennai. She had been visiting the hospital for dialysis, along with her attendant, for the past eight to nine years. With both her sons settled abroad and no one else to take care of the old lady, except the caretaker, like many others, she was also trapped in Kolathur, with no clue of how to deal with the situation.

In this desperate situation, Mahadevi reached out to Santa Kumar, whom she knew well at the hospital. He had even shared his visiting card with her in case of any emergency, but she had misplaced it. Thankfully, she had the number of the hospital's emergency unit saved, and so, made a call there to seek help to get out of this situation.

Since this was not a medical emergency and a one-of-a-kind request of disaster management, the emergency ambulance team was unsure what decision should be taken. Since the old lady had mentioned Santa's name during the call, the team approached him, and after discussing the matter with higher authorities, it was concluded that the lady and her caretaker should be rescued at the earliest.

Without any delay, a team of two to three staff members left for Kolathur in an ambulance and safely brought the old lady and her caretaker to the hospital. They were given shelter in the hospital, proving that in times of dire need, Apollo is always by your side.

Story 43

Committed to Caring

Apollo Main Hospital, Greams Road, Chennai

IN 2021, PRITAM BABU ACCOMPANIED HIS FRIEND TO APOLLO Main Hospital, Greams Road, Chennai for an out-patient consultation. While making his way to find a seat, Pritam Babu got injured by hitting a wall-mounted hand sanitizer and his shirt was torn.

The hospital's general manager happened to notice this incident during his routine round. At once, he approached Pritam Babu and offered him first aid, though thankfully, there was no serious injury, other than the torn shirt. The attendant was taken to the emergency unit and the on-duty staff member, Padmanabhan, and his supervisor, Kanniyappan, assisted in giving him a precautionary shot of the tetanus vaccine with the help of the emergency staff.

Meanwhile, the attendant and the patient were aided by the team throughout the out-patient consultation. The general manager informed the housekeeping team and instructed them to look for and remove any sharp objects from public areas, which could lead to minor accidents like the one with Pritam Babu.

Soon after the medical procedure got over, Mr Vijay, the linen team supervisor, offered Pritam Babu a brand-new shirt. This gesture was a complete surprise, and the two friends thanked the entire team, and especially, the general manager for going out of his way to make up for a small incident. A routine visit to the out-patient department left them with memories for a lifetime.

Story 44

A Camp with a Heart

Apollo Speciality Hospitals, Trichy

THE APOLLO SPECIALITY TEAM, TRICHY BECAME THE FIRST corporate hospital to join hands with government schemes for the deprived. Under the Rashtriya Bal Swasth Karyakram (RBSK), a beneficial scheme of the union government, the team held a camp from 1 April 2022 to 25 April 2022 for the diagnosis and treatment of congenital heart diseases, in the delta regions around Trichy.

The aim of this camp was to spread awareness about this disease and conduct screening and required treatment for the needy. Lesser-known facts about congenital heart diseases, which affect the target group from zero to eighteen years, were shared during the camp. Parents and children were educated on the importance of early management.

During the camp, a total of fifty-five children were diagnosed, out of which eighteen required immediate intervention. Under the scheme and the volunteered social service of Apollo, diagnosis, surgery and treatment were offered free of cost to all eighteen patients. The unit head, along with the deputy general manager and medical administrator, participated in the camp from day one with full support and cooperation. Right from picking up the patients from their home to providing them accommodation, food and complete treatment, the Apollo staff looked after every minute detail.

The admission of the patients began, and according to the schedule, all eighteen surgeries were conducted successfully. After surgery, the patients, along with their family members, were given proper counselling and were informed about post-surgical care.

Apollo Speciality Hospitals, Trichy was honoured with an award for their exemplary service under the Ayushman Bharat Pradhan Mantri Jan Arogya Yojna by the commissioner. Being the only corporate hospital to have received this honour, they have inspired other hospitals as well to come forward for a good cause.

Story 45

The Precious Gift

Apollo Speciality Hospitals, Trichy

A SEVENTY-NINE-YEAR-OLD LADY, VIMLABAI, WAS BROUGHT to Apollo Speciality Hospital, Trichy in October 2021. She had multiple ruptures, and Dr Arun suggested surgical intervention. But when the old lady was asked to remove her gold earrings for the procedure, she flatly refused. The earrings were a fiftieth-anniversary gift from her departed husband, and she had never taken them off.

After much coaxing and counselling, she took off the earrings, with strict instructions to keep them safe. Her surgery was successful, and as soon as Vimlabai regained consciousness, the first thing she enquired about was her pair of gold studs. But unfortunately, despite extra safety, one of her earrings was found missing. She burst into tears.

Housekeeping staff member Sabarunisha launched a thorough hunt for the missing earring but could not find it. Vimlabai was in deep sorrow, and on the day of her discharge, it was a great challenge for her attendants to lift her spirits and convince her to move home, taking one earring only.

The staff did not give up their search, and even before Vimlabai reached home, she received the news that the earring had been found. Her joy knew no bounds! The zeal and effort put in by the Apollo staff to ensure every patient's health and happiness prove the quote, 'Seek, and you shall find.'

Story 46

Caring Beyond Borders

Apollo Speciality Hospitals, OMR

IN SEPTEMBER 2022, TWENTY-YEAR-OLD JUBIN KHAN BROUGHT his father Imran Khan all the way from Bangladesh to Apollo Speciality Hospitals, OMR, Chennai, and he was admitted under Dr Joy Varghese, for treatment for a fast-spreading brain tumour.

Despite the best of treatment, doctors knew Imran would not survive. In addition to his tumour, the patient had also contracted COVID. Jubin was not only stressed, but also a bit lost because of the language barrier in a new country.

To his relief, he met one of Apollo's housekeeping staff members, Bikash Kumar. He was from Calcutta, knew their native language, and thus, they formed a bond and Bikash volunteered to be Jubin's translator. A few days later, Imran passed away, and Jubin had a new challenge to face. The government's COVID regulations did not permit him to take his deceased father's body back to his hometown in Bangladesh for the last rituals.

Jubin was clueless and heartbroken at the thought of not honouring his father with the last rituals. Nor did he have the money to hire a private plane back to Bangladesh. Bikash once again helped him out. He took a day's leave and obtained permission from the authorities to conduct Imran's last rites within the limits of the Chennai Corporation. He accompanied Jubin to his father's funeral and stood by him till the last moment.

Even though fate cannot be controlled, the Apollo family makes sure to do the best they can to serve their patients and their families.

Story 47

A Fond Farewell

Apollo Speciality Hospitals, OMR

HAVING THE PRIVILEGE TO WITNESS FOUR GENERATIONS grow in front of him, M.S. Anandswaroop had lived a happy life. But now he was old and suffering from multiple conditions, including lung cancer, brain metastasis and coronary artery disease. He was admitted to the hospital under the care of Dr Vijaya Raghavan in a state of emergency, just a couple of days before his birthday.

Considering his condition, the family knew it would be his last birthday celebration. They had planned a grand event at home, but now that Anandswaroop was in hospital, their preparations had come to nought. All they could hope for was his peaceful passing. With a heavy heart, his relatives signed the consent form and sat outside his room.

During her daily rounds, Nursing Head Ms Jeyarani spotted them and learnt of the situation. She instantly had an idea. Though nothing much could be done to improve Aanandswaroop's condition, the staff could at least put in the effort to celebrate the man's birthday.

She got in touch with the Manager on Duty Ms Nancy, and in no time, all the arrangements were done. A special cake was baked, and all his family members and close ones were invited to join the celebration. Since it was not certain if the patient would live for another day, the celebration was done on the day itself. Though Anandswaroop was unconscious, tears of happiness and contentment rolled down his eyes when he heard his great-grandchildren sing 'Happy Birthday' for him.

He bid a final adieu to the world within a couple of days. His family was extremely grateful for the kind gesture, and even today, they make it a point to look up the staff from time to time.

Story 48

Saying it with Roses

Apollo Cancer Centre, Teynampet

An aspiring ballet dancer, twelve-year-old Canadian Melinda Rose received a devastating piece of news—she had Askin's tumour, a rare type of blood cancer. Her condition was grave, and the doctors predicted that she had a couple of weeks at the most. But Melinda chose not to give up. She not only uplifted her own spirits, but also counselled several young cancer victims around the world. Her sheer spirit extended her life by another three years, and she left the world with the optimistic slogan, 'Cancer is not the end of life. It is just the beginning.'

Every year, 22 September is celebrated as 'World Rose Day' in remembrance of Melinda Rose. The Apollo Cancer Centre, Teynampet also celebrates this day every year. In 2022, the Centre arranged to rejoice and cheer up every cancer survivor with a rose as a sign of love offered by famous Tamil actor Silambarasan T.R. He was invited on the special demand of a girl patient as a long-awaited wish of meeting the 'little superstar'.

Silambarasan, along with the other team members of the Centre, made the day a memorable one for the tiny fighters by offering them rose-shaped candies and chocolates. The guests at the paediatric ward were surprised and delighted. Seeing the happy smiles on the little one's faces brought joy to the hearts of the entire staff of the Centre.

Story 49

Read This and Smile

Apollo Gleneagles Hospital, Kolkata

MEDHA BISWAS, A REGULAR AT APOLLO GLENEAGLES Hospital, Kolkata for her chemotherapy sessions, had built a strong bond with the doctors and staff Dr P.N. Mahapatra, Dr Animesh Shah, Guest Relations Executive Ms Sharmila, and nursing staff Sister Yasira Khatun, Sister Rupinder Singh, Brother Ratnadeep and Ananya Chatterjee had become more like family to her, since her husband was old and her only son was settled in the US.

A tough lady, Medha fought cancer with a smile on her face and a book in her hand. Books seemed to be her best friend, and never left her side. During a conversation with Guest Relations Executive Ms Sharmila, Medha told her about one particular book that she wanted to read but was unable to find. It was called *Conundrum*, and it revealed several interesting facts behind Netaji's death.

In June, Medha was to have her last chemotherapy session. It was a special day, and the staff wanted to make it even more special for their bibliophile patient. The guest relations team bought *Conundrum* and wrapped it beautifully for Medha.

When Medha came to bid goodbye to the team, they handed her the surprise. She was speechless at their thoughtful gesture and thanked them profusely.

Story 50

The Sunday Phone Call

Apollo Hospitals, Ahmedabad

A RATHER QUIET SUNDAY. SUDDENLY, THE LOUD RING OF THE phone broke the silence at Apollo Hospitals, Ahmedabad.

The on-duty staff member, Prakash Solanki, picked up the call and was startled to hear the quivering voice of a lady who sounded very old. She had called to request for a health certificate and some specific health records.

Calming her down, Prakash asked her for details. She told him she was eighty-three, visually challenged, and had been a patient of Dr Naresh. He tried explaining to her that it was Sunday, and the concerned authorities were all on leave, but the lady was adamant that she needed the documents urgently. Finally, Prakash assured her he would do his best to help.

After putting the phone down, he, along with two other staff members, Yogesh Nagar and Parth Prajapati, got down to work. The team got in touch with the head of the respective department and sought permission to access the authorities' cabin to search for the requested documents. Permission was granted, and the team began the hunt for the documents the old lady had asked for.

It took a lot of time and effort, but the papers were located and mailed to the lady, who thanked the team a million times for putting in the extra effort and adhering to her urgent request.

Acknowledgements

THIS BOOK IS A TRIBUTE TO THE GENEROUS SPIRIT OF OUR staff, who went beyond the call of duty to do more than provide medical care. Their simple acts of thoughtfulness, often presented as sweet surprises, touched our patients and their families to the core and made unforgettable memories. Each of the stories in these pages reflects Apollo's abiding belief in healing with a human touch.

The completion of this undertaking could not have been possible without the participation and assistance of numerous people. While it may not be possible to name them all, we would like to express our deep appreciation and indebtedness particularly to the following:

Our beloved chairman and visionary, Dr Prathap C. Reddy, who has instilled in us the value of kindness and taught us to go the extra mile.

Our Vice Chairpersons Dr Preetha Reddy and Ms Shobana Kamineni, Managing Director Ms Suneeta Reddy, Joint Managing Director Dr Sangita Reddy and President Dr K Hari Prasad, for being our guiding lights and inspiring us at every step. We most certainly could not dream of having better mentors to lead us by example.

Our unit heads, service excellence leads, quality and operation heads, our incredible medical and nursing and administrative team, and the entire marketing and public relations team for making this book possible. Their contributions are sincerely appreciated and gratefully acknowledged.

Rakesh Chander of HarperCollins and Shubhra Krishan: thank you for collating the stories and shaping them beautifully.

> *'Not all of us can do great things. But we can do small things with great love.'*
>
> – Mother Teresa

About Apollo Hospitals

Apollo Hospitals has been redefining healthcare since 1983. The establishment of the Apollo Hospitals Group began with a dream to make world-class healthcare accessible and affordable to every Indian. Its pioneering journey has seen the group grow from the first modern hospital in Chennai to Asia's foremost integrated healthcare services provider.

Recognized as the architect of private healthcare in India, Apollo Hospitals is today present in every link of the healthcare chain, with 12,000 beds across seventy-four hospitals, 4,500+ pharmacies, 120+ primary care centres, over 720 diagnostic centres and 500+ telemedicine centres across thirteen countries.

As an integrated healthcare service provider, the Apollo Group encompasses a Global Projects Consultancy capability, over fifteen medical education centres, and a research foundation with a focus on global clinical trials, epidemiological studies, stem cell and genetic research. The future-ready group has always stayed ahead of the curve by investing in the latest medical technologies such as halcyon and proton therapy.

Apollo Hospitals was among the first healthcare providers to recognize the potential of and implement technologies like artificial intelligence (AI), robotics and data analytics to provide high-quality healthcare for India's vast population of 1.3 billion. They kickstarted a digital revolution in healthcare by connecting with the common man via their Apollo 24/7 App.

With every new hospital open, we set new benchmarks in quality control, processes and infrastructure. The Indraprastha Apollo Hospitals was the first to get the coveted Joint Commission International (JCI) accreditation in the country in 2005. Apollo Hospitals took the lead in helping the government set up the National Accreditation Board for Hospitals and Healthcare Providers (NABH) and draft the standards that hospitals across the country abide by today. The group includes eight JCI-accredited hospitals and twenty-three NABH accredited hospitals, a testament to the world-class quality of care at one-tenth of the cost abroad. One of the most respected healthcare institutions in the world, Apollo Hospitals is also a beacon of hope for medical value travellers from across the globe.

At the core of Apollo's patient-centric culture is tender loving care (TLC), the magic that inspires hope among its patients. Cutting-edge technologies have enabled us to deliver personalized and precise treatments that boost patients' confidence and trust in their doctors. Our dedicated centres of excellence (CoEs) cover super-specialities such as cardiac sciences, oncology, transplant, orthopaedics, neuroscience and emergency. These CoEs are marked by a focus on world-class clinical outcomes, comparable to the best in the West, safety through systems and protocols, the expertise of over 8,000 specialists in fifty-five specialties, and the trust of millions of patients.

The stories are all real and to ensure patient privacy and confidentiality, we have changed the patient names and other personal details. The changed/fictitious names may bear resemblance to others but have no connection with the stories in this book.

Apollo Hospitals also confirms that all mandated COVID-19 protocols and regulations prevalent at different points in time were duly adhered to while our team members were offering tender, loving care to our patients. All processes including vaccination at home as necessitated by patient's condition were adhered to as per the related clinical and non-clinical protocols.

At no time was any patient's clinical care or the safety of any patient's attendant or even staff put at risk.

30 Years *of*

HarperCollins *Publishers* India

At HarperCollins, we believe in telling the best stories and finding the widest possible readership for our books in every format possible. We started publishing 30 years ago; a great deal has changed since then, but what has remained constant is the passion with which our authors write their books, the love with which readers receive them, and the sheer joy and excitement that we as publishers feel in being a part of the publishing process.

Over the years, we've had the pleasure of publishing some of the finest writing from the subcontinent and around the world, and some of the biggest bestsellers in India's publishing history. Our books and authors have won a phenomenal range of awards, and we ourselves have been named Publisher of the Year the greatest number of times. But nothing has meant more to us than the fact that millions of people have read the books we published, and somewhere, a book of ours might have made a difference.

As we step into our fourth decade, we go back to that one word – a word which has been a driving force for us all these years.

Read.

Harper Collins · 4th · HARPER PERENNIAL · HARPER BUSINESS · HARPER BLACK · हार्पर हिन्दी

HarperCollins *Children'sBooks* · HARPER DESIGN · HARPER VANTAGE · Harper Sport